BREAST CANCER
ALERT

How to be tougher to defeat a tough disease

By

Mary J. Douglas

TABLE OF CONTENTS

INTRODUCTION

Eugenia Adams was a vivacious, energetic woman who had always taken good care of her health. She ate healthily, exercised consistently, and went for regular check-ups with her doctor. So when she felt a lump in her breast during a self-examination, she was understandably alarmed.

At first, Eugenia attempted to ignore the lump, expecting that it would go away on its own. But it didn't, and ultimately she arranged an appointment with her doctor. After a series of tests and scans, Eugenia received the news that no woman wants to hear: she had breast cancer.

Eugenia was devastated. She had always thought of cancer as something that occurred to other people, not to her. But now it was her reality, and she had to face it head-on.

Over the next six months, Eugenia had a series of therapies for her breast cancer, including surgery, chemotherapy, and radiation. It was a challenging period for her, both physically and mentally. But through it all, Eugenia stayed resolute to fight cancer and emerge stronger for it.

With the support of her family, friends, and medical team, Eugenia navigated the ups and downs of breast cancer treatment. She learned how to manage the physical side effects of treatment, and how to cope with the emotional toll of a cancer diagnosis.

And despite the challenges she experienced, Eugenia never lost her sense of hope. She stayed devoted to living her life to the fullest, and to motivating other women to do the same.

Now, as a breast cancer survivor, Eugenia is sharing her story with others. She believes that by sharing her experience, she might assist other women who are facing a breast cancer diagnosis to feel less alone and to find the fortitude and courage to fight the disease with everything they've got.

Chapter One

UNDERSTANDING BREAST CANCER

WHAT IS BREAST CANCER

Breast cancer is a type of cancer that arises in the cells of the breast tissue. It develops when cells in the breast begin to grow out of control, causing a tumor that may be felt as a lump or seen on mammography. Breast cancer can occur in both men and women, but it is considerably more common in women. There are various kinds of breast cancer, including ductal carcinoma in situ (DCIS), invasive ductal carcinoma (IDC), and invasive lobular carcinoma (ILC).

DCIS is a non-invasive kind of breast cancer that is restricted to the milk ducts, while IDC and ILC are invasive types of breast cancer that have moved beyond the milk ducts into the surrounding glandular or breast tissue.

Breast cancer can cause a range of symptoms, including a lump or thickening in the breast or underarm area, changes in the size or shape of the breast, nipple discharge or inversion, and skin changes such as redness, scaliness, or puckering.

Treatment for breast cancer often comprises of a combination of surgery, chemotherapy, radiation therapy, and/or hormone therapy. The type and duration of treatment will depend on the stage and type of breast cancer, as well as the patient's overall health and preferences.

Breast cancer is a serious and possibly life-threatening disease, but with early identification and prompt treatment, many people can successfully fight the disease and go on to live long healthy lives.

TYPES OF BREAST CANCER

There are various forms of breast cancer, which can be broadly categorized into two categories: non-invasive (also called in situ) and invasive (also called infiltrating) breast cancer.

1. Non-Invasive Breast Cancer

This is also known as in situ breast cancer, refers to abnormal cells that are contained inside the milk ducts (ductal carcinoma in situ or DCIS) or lobules (lobular carcinoma in situ or LCIS) of the breast. These cells have not spread to neighboring breast tissue or other regions of the body, making them easier to treat and cure.

DCIS is the most frequent type of non-invasive breast cancer, accounting for around 20% of all breast cancer cases. It is commonly discovered through mammography, which can indicate tiny clusters of calcifications in the breast. DCIS is considered a pre-cancerous condition, as there is a possibility that the abnormal cells could someday grow into invasive breast cancer if left untreated.

LCIS is less prevalent than DCIS and is usually not identified with a mammogram. Instead, it is commonly detected inadvertently after a biopsy or surgery for another illness. LCIS is also considered a pre-cancerous disease, as it raises the risk of developing invasive breast cancer later in life.

2. Invasive Breast Cancer

This is a form of cancer that starts in the milk ducts or lobules of the breast and has gone beyond the initial site into the surrounding breast tissue. This type of breast cancer is more aggressive and has a higher risk of spreading to other parts of the body than non-invasive breast cancer.

Invasive ductal carcinoma (IDC) is the most frequent kind of invasive breast cancer, accounting for around 80% of all occurrences. IDC originates in the milk ducts of the breast and can spread to other regions of the body if left untreated. Symptoms of IDC may include a lump in the breast, changes in breast shape or size, nipple discharge, or changes in the skin of the breast.

Invasive lobular carcinoma (ILC) is less prevalent than IDC, accounting for roughly 10% to 15% of all invasive breast malignancies. ILC starts in the milk-producing glands (lobules) of the breast and can also spread to other regions of the body if left untreated. Symptoms of ILC may include a thickness or fullness in the breast, changes in breast form or size, or nipple discharge.

- Invasive ductal carcinoma (IDC)

Invasive ductal carcinoma (IDC) is the most prevailing kind of breast cancer, accounting for almost 80% of all invasive breast cancers. IDC arises when cancer cells that have developed in the milk ducts of the breast burst through the duct walls and infect the surrounding breast tissue. The symptoms of IDC might vary but may include a lump or thickening in the breast or armpit, changes in breast size or shape, skin dimpling or puckering, nipple inversion or discharge, or redness or scaling of the breast surface.

- Invasive lobular carcinoma (ILC)

Invasive lobular carcinoma (ILC) is a kind of breast cancer that develops in the lobules or milk-producing glands of the breast. ILC accounts for roughly 10% to 15% of all breast cancers.

The signs of ILC can include a thickening or lump in the breast tissue, changes in the texture or appearance of the breast skin, or nipple alterations such as inversion or discharge. However, some persons with ILC may not suffer any obvious symptoms.

ILC tends to grow and spread more diffusely than other types of breast cancer, which can make it more difficult to identify and treat. It may also be more likely to arise in both breasts at the same time or to reoccur following therapy.

Inflammatory Breast Cancer (IBC)

Inflammatory breast cancer (IBC) is an uncommon but severe form of breast cancer that accounts for roughly 1% to 5% of all breast cancer cases. IBC develops when cancer cells block the lymphatic veins on the surface of the breast, causing the breast to become red, swollen, and warm to the touch. The skin of the breast may also appear thick, pitted, or ridged, with a texture akin to that of an orange peel.

IBC tends to develop more rapidly than other types of breast cancer, and may not create a distinct lump that can be felt during a breast exam. This can make it more difficult to identify and diagnose, which might delay treatment and lead to a poorer prognosis.

Triple-Negative Breast Cancer (TNBC)

Triple-negative breast cancer (TNBC) is a kind of breast cancer that is negative for estrogen receptor (ER), progesterone receptor (PR), and human epidermal growth factor receptor 2 (HER2). This means that TNBC does not react to hormonal therapy or targeted therapies that are designed to prevent the proliferation of cancer cells that rely on these receptors.

TNBC accounts for roughly 10% to 20% of all breast cancer cases and tends to be more aggressive and has a poorer prognosis than other kinds of breast cancer. TNBC is also more likely to arise in younger women, African American women, and women with a BRCA1 gene mutation.

The signs of TNBC can include a lump or thickening in the breast or armpit, changes in breast size or form, skin dimpling or puckering, nipple inversion or discharge, or redness or scaling of the breast skin.

HER2-Positive Breast Cancer

HER2-positive breast cancer is a kind of breast cancer that tests positive for a specific protein called human epidermal growth factor receptor 2 (HER2). This protein plays a function in the growth and division of cells, and when it is overexpressed in breast cancer cells, it can cause the disease to grow and spread more quickly.

HER2-positive breast cancer accounts for roughly 20% of all breast cancer cases and tends to be more aggressive and has a poorer prognosis than HER2-negative breast cancer. HER2-positive breast cancer is also more likely to occur in younger women and women with a family history of breast cancer.

The signs of HER2-positive breast cancer can include a lump or thickening in the breast or armpit, changes in breast size or form, skin dimpling or puckering, nipple inversion or discharge, or redness or scaling of the breast surface.

Male Breast Cancer

Male breast cancer is an uncommon but deadly form of cancer that arises when malignant cells originate in the breast tissue of men. Although breast cancer is more often associated with women, men can also develop the disease. It is anticipated that roughly 1 in 1,000 males may develop breast cancer in their lifetime.

The signs of male breast cancer can include a lump or swelling in the breast tissue, nipple discharge, or changes in the look of the nipple or breast skin. However, many men with breast cancer may not experience any visible symptoms, which can make early detection and diagnosis more complicated.

Paget's Disease Of the Nipple

Paget's disease of the nipple is an uncommon form of breast cancer that affects the skin of the nipple and the areola (the dark region surrounding the nipple). It is thought that Paget's illness accounts for only approximately 1% to 4% of all breast cancer cases.

The symptoms of Paget's disease of the nipple can include itching, redness, scaling, or peeling of the nipple or areola, as well as a discharge from the nipple. These symptoms can be similar to those of other skin illnesses, such as eczema or dermatitis, which can make diagnosis more complicated. Paget's disease of the nipple is typically associated with underlying breast cancer, which may or may not be identified in imaging studies.

Chapter Two

CAUSES ÀND RISK FACTORS OF CANCER

Cancer can be caused by a variety of reasons, including genetic changes, exposure to carcinogens (such as cigarette smoke, radiation, and certain chemicals), viruses and infections, and lifestyle factors (such as food, physical activity, and alcohol intake).

However, it's important to emphasize that not all occurrences of cancer are avoidable, and having one or more risk factors does not guarantee that a person will acquire cancer. Many malignancies are also impacted by random chance and other elements that are not yet fully understood.

It's crucial to maintain a healthy lifestyle and prevent exposure to recognized carcinogens to lessen the risk of acquiring cancer. Additionally, routine cancer screenings and early identification can enhance treatment outcomes and raise the odds of survival.

Genetic Mutations

Genetic mutations are variations in the DNA sequence that can raise the risk of developing cancer. Some genetic mutations are inherited from a parent, while others occur spontaneously during a person's lifespan.

Inherited genetic alterations, such as mutations in the BRCA1 and BRCA2 genes, can dramatically increase the chance of developing breast, ovarian, and other types of cancer. These mutations are relatively rare, but those who carry them have a substantially higher chance of developing cancer than the general population.

Spontaneous genetic mutations can also arise over a person's lifespan due to exposure to environmental variables, such as radiation and certain chemicals, as well as other factors that are not yet fully understood. These mutations can accumulate over time and raise the chance of developing cancer. it's crucial to note that not all persons with these mutations will develop cancer.

Genetic testing can assist identify individuals who may be at increased risk of developing cancer due to genetic mutations. For people who are determined to have a genetic mutation, there may be possibilities for risk-reducing interventions, such as greater surveillance, preventive surgery, and/or chemoprevention.

Environmental Factors

Environmental factors can also play a role in increasing the risk of breast cancer. These environmental factors can include exposure to various chemicals, radiation, and other environmental toxins.

One example of an environmental factor that has been related to an elevated risk of breast cancer is exposure to endocrine-disrupting chemicals. These compounds, which can be found in certain pesticides, plastics, and other items, can mimic the effects of hormones in the body and disrupt normal hormone function. This can lead to an increased risk of breast cancer, as some breast tumors are hormone-sensitive.

Radiation exposure, particularly throughout childhood and adolescence, has also been related to an increased risk of breast cancer. This can involve exposure to medical radiation, such as radiation therapy for Hodgkin's lymphoma, as well as exposure to environmental radiation, such as from nuclear accidents. Other environmental factors that have been related to an increased risk of breast cancer include exposure to some air pollutants, such as benzene and polycyclic aromatic hydrocarbons

(PAHs), as well as exposure to certain metals such as cadmium

Lifestyle Factors

There is evidence to show that certain lifestyle variables can raise a person's risk of acquiring breast cancer. Some of the lifestyle factors that have been related to an increased risk of breast cancer include:

- Obesity

Being overweight or obese has been related to an increased risk of breast cancer, particularly in postmenopausal women.

- Physical inactivity

Lack of regular physical activity has been associated with an increased risk of breast cancer, presumably due to its effect on hormone levels.

- Alcohol consumption

Drinking alcohol, even in moderate doses, has been connected with an increased risk of breast cancer.

- Smoking

Smoking has been associated with an increased risk of breast cancer, particularly in younger women.

- Diet

A diet high in saturated and trans fats, red and processed meats, and low in fruits and vegetables has been associated with an increased risk of breast cancer.

Reproductive History

Reproductive history is a well-established risk factor for breast cancer. Women who have specific reproductive characteristics may have a higher risk of having breast cancer than those who do not. Some of the reproductive factors that have been related to an increased risk of breast cancer include:

- Age at first menstrual period

Women who started menstruating at an early age (before the age of 12) had a slightly increased chance of developing breast cancer than those who started menstruating at a later age.

- Age at menopause

Women who experience menopause at a later age (beyond the age of 55) have a slightly higher chance of developing breast cancer than those who experience menopause at an earlier age.

- Pregnancy and childbirth

Women who have never had children or who had their first kid after the age of 30 may have a slightly higher chance of developing breast cancer than those who had their first child at a younger age.

- Breastfeeding

Women who breastfeed their children may have a slightly decreased chance of developing breast cancer than those who do not.

- Hormone replacement therapy

The use of hormone replacement therapy (HRT) for menopausal symptoms has been related to an increased risk of breast cancer, particularly in women who take it for a lengthy period.

Chapter Three

SCREENING DIAGNOSIS AND STAGING OF BREAST CANCER

Screening And Diagnosis

Breast cancer screening includes testing a woman's breasts for cancer before there are signs or symptoms of the disease. All women need to be informed by their healthcare practitioner about the best screening choices for them. When you are taught about the advantages and dangers of screening and decide with your health care provider if screening is best for you and if so, when to have it. This is called informed and shared decision-making.

Although breast cancer screening cannot prevent breast cancer, it can help discover breast cancer early, when it is simpler to cure. Talk to your doctor about which breast cancer screening tests are suitable for you, and when you should have them.

Various forms of breast cancer screenings can be used to identify breast cancer, including:

Mammography

Mammography is a sort of breast cancer screening that uses X-rays to identify breast cancer before a lump can be felt. During mammography, the breast is squeezed between two plates, and an X-ray image is taken. Mammograms can reveal very minor abnormalities in the breast, including regions of calcification and small cancers that may not be detected during a physical exam.

Mammograms are advised for women starting at age 40, or earlier for women with a family history of breast cancer. Women should continue to receive frequent mammograms as long as they are in good health. Mammograms are routinely done every one to two years.

While mammograms are an excellent technique for detecting breast cancer early, they are not perfect. False positives, where mammography suggests the presence of cancer when there is none, can occur. False negatives, where mammography fails to detect cancer that is present, can also occur. Additionally, mammography may not detect all kinds of breast cancer, particularly in individuals with dense breast tissue.

Clinical Breast Examination

A clinical breast examination is a physical examination of the breast performed by a healthcare provider. During a clinical breast exam, the healthcare professional will search for any abnormalities in the breast, such as lumps, thickness, or changes in the skin or nipple. They will also feel the breast tissue to look for any abnormalities.

Clinical breast exams are often done in conjunction with a mammogram and may be advised for women who are at high risk for breast cancer, or for women who have symptoms such as breast soreness or a new lump. Clinical breast checks may also be recommended for women who are unable to get a mammogram, such as pregnant women or women with breast implants.

While clinical breast exams are a useful tool for detecting breast cancer, they are not ideal. Small tumors or abnormalities may be missed during a clinical breast exam. Additionally, some breast tumors may not present any symptoms or changes that may be felt during a physical exam.

Breast Self-Examination

Breast self-examination (BSE) is a simple and efficient approach for women to become familiar with their breasts and to notice any changes that may arise. By practicing BSE periodically, women can become more aware of their breast tissue and recognize any abnormalities that may develop, such as lumps, edema, or changes in the skin.

To perform BSE, it is vital to first become familiar with the typical look and feel of your breasts. This can be done by looking at your breasts in the mirror and feeling them with your hands. Note any changes in the size, shape, or look of your breasts, as well as any changes in the texture or feel of the breast tissue.

To execute BSE, follow these steps:

- Lie down on your back with a pillow or towel under your right shoulder.
- Behind your head, place your right hand
- Use the pads of your left fingers to feel for lumps or other changes in your right breast. Use a circular motion, starting at the outer edge of the breast and going toward the nipple.
- Use gentle, medium, and strong pressure to feel different depths of the breast tissue.
- Move around the breast in an up-and-down movement until you have felt the entire breast.
- Repeat these techniques on your left breast.

It is crucial to conduct BSE periodically, ideally once a month. By doing so, you can become more comfortable with the normal look and feel of your breasts and spot any changes early on. If you observe any changes or anomalies in your breast tissue, it is crucial to inform your healthcare professional as soon as possible. Remember, early identification is important in the successful treatment of breast cancer.

Breast Magnetic Resonance Imaging (MRI)

Magnetic resonance imaging (MRI) is a method of breast cancer screening that employs a powerful magnet and radio waves to obtain detailed images of the breast tissue. MRI screening is generally advised for women who have an elevated risk of breast cancer, such as those with a family history of the disease or those who have tested positive for particular genetic abnormalities.

During an MRI screening, the patient lies on their stomach on a customized table that slides into the MRI machine. The equipment creates images of the breast tissue, which are then evaluated by a radiologist to check for any abnormalities, such as tumors or areas of increased blood flow.

MRI screening is more sensitive than mammography in detecting breast cancer, particularly in women with dense breast tissue. However, it is also more likely to provide false-positive results, which can lead to unneeded biopsies or other operations. For this reason, MRI screening is often used in conjunction with mammography and other breast cancer screening modalities, rather than as a substitute.

DIAGNOSIS

The diagnosis of breast cancer often involves a combination of imaging tests, such as mammography, ultrasound, or MRI, and a biopsy, which involves removing a tiny sample of breast tissue for study.

If imaging studies show the presence of cancer, a biopsy will be conducted to confirm the diagnosis. There are various types of biopsies that can be conducted, including:

Fine-Needle Aspiration Biopsy

Fine needle aspiration biopsy (FNAB) is a form of biopsy that is used to analyze breast abnormalities, such as lumps or masses, that are found on imaging tests, such as mammography, ultrasound, or MRI. FNAB includes using a tiny needle to take a small sample of cells or fluid from the breast tissue for analysis.

During an FNAB, the patient normally lies down on their back or sits upright, and the skin above the area to be biopsied is cleansed and numbed with a local anesthetic. A thin needle is then introduced into the breast tissue, usually with the aid of ultrasonography or mammography, and a small sample of cells or fluid is extracted into the needle. The needle is then withdrawn, and the sample is transported to a laboratory for analysis by a pathologist.

FNAB is a minimally invasive treatment that can be performed swiftly and easily in an outpatient setting. It is often less painful and has a shorter recovery time than other forms of biopsies, such as core needle biopsy or surgical biopsy. However, it may not produce enough tissue for a definitive diagnosis in some circumstances and may need to be followed up with more biopsies or imaging studies.

FNAB is most typically used to analyze breast lumps or masses that are suspected of malignancy in imaging studies. It can help to evaluate whether a lump is a benign cyst, a non-cancerous growth, or a dangerous tumor. If cancer is diagnosed, the pathologist can also determine the type of cancer and its characteristics, such as its stage and grade

Core Needle Biopsy

Core needle biopsy (CNB) is a form of biopsy that is used to analyze breast abnormalities, such as lumps or masses, that are found on imaging tests, such as mammography, ultrasound, or MRI. CNB entails utilizing a bigger needle to retrieve a tiny core of tissue from the breast for analysis.

During a CNB, the patient normally lies down on their back or sits upright, and the skin above the area to be biopsied is cleansed and numbed with a local anesthetic. A bigger needle, usually about the size of a pencil lead, is then pushed into the breast tissue, usually with the guidance of ultrasonography or mammography, and a small core of tissue is extracted. The needle is then withdrawn, and the sample is transported to a laboratory for analysis by a pathologist.

CNB is a minimally invasive technique that can be performed swiftly and easily in an outpatient setting. It gives a larger sample of tissue than fine needle aspiration biopsy (FNAB), which can help to provide a more definitive diagnosis. It is also less intrusive than surgical biopsy, which requires taking a bigger sample of breast tissue under general anesthesia.

CNB is most typically used to analyze breast lumps or masses that are suspected of malignancy in imaging studies. It can help to evaluate whether a lump is a benign cyst, a non-cancerous growth, or a dangerous tumor. If cancer is identified, the pathologist can also establish the type of cancer and its features, such as its stage and grade.

Vacuum-Assisted Biopsy

A vacuum-assisted biopsy is a minimally invasive method used to acquire a tissue sample from the breast for further investigation. This treatment is often performed to assist identify breast cancer or other breast problems.

During the surgery, a small incision is created in the skin of the breast, and a hollow probe is introduced into the incision. The probe employs suction to draw out a tiny tissue sample from the breast. The probe spins and takes many tissue samples from different angles to boost the accuracy of the diagnosis.

Vacuum-assisted biopsy is a safe and successful method that can be conducted in an outpatient environment under local anesthetic. The treatment normally takes roughly 30 to 60 minutes to complete, and the patient can go home the same day. After the biopsy, the tissue sample is transported to a laboratory for analysis. The results of the biopsy can assist establish if cancer is present, and if so, what form of breast cancer it is. This information is critical for formulating a suitable treatment plan

Surgical Biopsy

A surgical biopsy is a process in which a surgeon takes a sample of breast tissue for examination under a microscope. This sort of biopsy is often advised when imaging tests, such as mammography or ultrasound, show a questionable area of the breast that cannot be easily accessible with a needle biopsy.

There are two major forms of surgical biopsy: an open biopsy and a needle localization biopsy. An open biopsy includes creating an incision in the breast and removing a sample of tissue. A needle localization biopsy involves putting a small wire or needle into the breast to guide the surgeon to the area of concern.

A surgical biopsy is commonly done under local anesthetic with sedation or general anesthesia, and it may necessitate an overnight hospital stay. After the procedure, the tissue sample is transported to a laboratory for analysis. The results of the biopsy can assist establish if cancer is present, and if so, what form of breast cancer it is. This information is critical for formulating a suitable treatment plan.

While surgical biopsy is a more invasive process than a needle biopsy, it may be essential to collect a bigger or more representative tissue sample. Surgical biopsy is generally regarded safe, although as with any surgical operation, there is a risk of bleeding, infection, and other consequences.

It is crucial to review the risks and advantages of surgical biopsy with a healthcare provider and to ask any questions or express any concerns before the surgery. The healthcare professional can help choose which form of biopsy is most appropriate for the individual patient's situation.

BREAST CANCER STAGING

Breast cancer staging is a technique of describing the size and extent of the cancer and if it has progressed beyond the breast. Staging is significant because it helps select the best therapy options and provides a prognosis for the patient.

The most common staging procedure for breast cancer is the TNM staging system, which stands for

Tumor, Node, and Metastasis. The T category defines the size of the main tumor, the N category describes if cancer has migrated to surrounding lymph nodes, and the M category describes whether cancer has migrated to other organs, such as the lungs or liver.

The T category is separated into four stages, from T1 (small, confined tumor) to T4 (big, invasive tumor). The N category is separated into three stages, from N0 (no lymph node involvement) to N3 (severe lymph node involvement). The M category is separated into two stages, M0 (no distant metastasis) and M1 (distant metastasis present).

Based on the T, N, and M categories, breast cancer is assigned an overall stage from 0 to IV.

Stage 0 BreastCancer(Carcinoma in Situ)

Stage 0 breast cancer, also known as carcinoma in situ, refers to abnormal cells that are present within the milk ducts or lobules of the breast but have not migrated beyond those areas. Stage 0 breast cancer is considered non-invasive, meaning it has not yet expanded into surrounding breast tissue or spread to lymph nodes or other regions of the body.

Stage 0 breast cancer comes in two main forms namely ductal carcinoma in situ (DCIS) and lobular carcinoma in situ (LCIS). DCIS refers to aberrant cells that are confined to the milk ducts, while LCIS refers to abnormal cells that are confined to the lobules.

DCIS and LCIS are both regarded to be precancerous conditions because they have the potential to become invasive breast cancer if left untreated. However, they are also extremely curable, and the prognosis for stage 0 breast cancer is often very favorable.

Stage I Breast Cancer

Stage 1 breast cancer is invasive, meaning it has progressed beyond the milk ducts or lobules of the breast and into adjacent tissue. In stage 1 breast cancer, the tumor measures up to 2 centimeters in diameter and has not migrated to the lymph nodes or other regions of the body.

There are two subgroups of stage 1 breast cancer: stage 1A and stage 1B. In stage 1A, the tumor measures up to 2 cm in diameter and has not progressed beyond the breast. In stage 1B, either there is no tumor in the breast, but cancer cells are detected in the lymph nodes, or the tumor measures between 1 and 2 centimeters in diameter and has not progressed beyond the breast.

Stage 2 Breast Cancer

Stage 2 breast cancer is invasive cancer that has gone beyond the breast and adjacent lymph nodes but has not yet migrated to distant organs. There are two subgroups of stage 2 breast cancer, namely stage 2A and stage 2B.

In stage 2A, one of the following characteristics is met:

- The tumor measures between 2 and 5 centimeters in diameter and has spread to the adjacent lymph nodes.
- The tumor measures up to 2 centimeters in diameter but has migrated to the adjacent lymph nodes.

In stage 2B, one of the following characteristics is met:

- The tumor measures between 2 and 5 centimeters in diameter and has not spread to the adjacent lymph nodes.
- The tumor measures more than 5 cm in diameter but has not migrated to the adjacent lymph nodes.

Stage 3 Breast Cancer

Stage 3 breast cancer is an invasive cancer that has progressed beyond the breast and adjacent lymph nodes and has also expanded to the lymph nodes positioned above or below the collarbone. There are three subcategories of stage 3 breast cancer: stage 3A, stage 3B, and stage 3C.

In stage 3A, one of the following conditions is met:

- The tumor may be any size and has migrated to the adjacent lymph nodes that are clumped together or clinging to other tissues in the chest.
- The tumor is greater than 5 centimeters in diameter and has migrated to the adjacent lymph nodes.

In stage 3B, one of the following conditions is met:

- The tumor may be any size, and has spread to the skin of the breast or chest wall, causing swelling, redness, or ulcers.
- The tumor has spread to the chest wall or the skin of the breast, and may or may not have migrated to adjacent lymph nodes.
- The tumor may be any size and has progressed to the lymph nodes positioned above or below the collarbone.

In stage 3C, the tumor has spread to the lymph nodes positioned above or below the collarbone, and may or may not have expanded to the adjacent lymph nodes or the wall of the chest or skin of the breast.

Stage 4 Breast Cancer

Stage 4 breast cancer, also known as metastatic breast cancer, is an advanced stage of breast cancer in which the disease has gone beyond the breast and adjacent lymph nodes to other organs in the body, such as the lungs, liver, bones, or brain.

In stage 4 breast cancer, the cancer may be discovered in one or more distant areas of the body. This is also known as secondary or metastatic cancer. Stage 4 breast cancer is generally incurable, however, it can be treated to help stop the spread of the disease and manage symptoms.

Chapter Four

TREATMENT OPTIONS FOR BREAST CANCER

The treatment options for breast cancer rely on various aspects, including the stage and type of disease, as well as the patient's overall health and personal preferences. The most prevalent treatment options for breast cancer include:

SURGERY

Breast cancer surgery is a popular treatment option for early-stage breast cancer. The goal of breast cancer surgery is to remove the tumor and surrounding tissue while preserving as much of the breast as feasible. There are various forms of breast cancer surgery, including:

Lumpectomy

Lumpectomy is a type of breast cancer surgery that includes removing the tumor and a small amount of surrounding tissue while leaving the rest of the breast intact. It is also known as breast-conserving surgery or partial mastectomy.

A lumpectomy is often used to treat early-stage breast cancer that has not progressed beyond the breast. The goal of a lumpectomy is to remove the cancer while preserving as much of the breast as feasible. This can help to maintain the natural contour and look of the breast.

A lumpectomy is normally conducted under general anesthesia, which means the patient will be sleeping during the procedure. During the procedure, the surgeon will make a small incision in the breast and remove the tumor and a small quantity of surrounding tissue. The incision is subsequently closed with stitches or surgical tape.

Mastectomy

Mastectomy is a surgical technique to remove all or part of the breast tissue. It is primarily performed as a treatment for breast cancer, but it may also be done as a preventive strategy for women who are at high risk of getting breast cancer.

There are various distinct forms of mastectomy, including:

- Total mastectomy or simple mastectomy

This entails the removal of the entire breast, including the nipple and areola.

- Modified radical mastectomy

This comprises the removal of the entire breast, as well as the axillary lymph nodes beneath the arm.

- Radical mastectomy

This involves the removal of the entire breast, as well as the chest muscles and axillary lymph nodes.

- Skin-sparing mastectomy

This entails the removal of the breast tissue, but not the skin overlaying the breast. This allows for breast reconstruction to be done more simply.

- Nipple-sparing mastectomy

This entails the removal of the breast tissue, but not the nipple or areola. This also allows for breast reconstruction to be done more readily.

The type of mastectomy that is recommended will depend on various criteria, including the size and location of the tumor, the stage of the disease, and the patient's overall health and preferences.

After a mastectomy, breast reconstruction may be done to restore the look of the breast. This can be done using implants or the patient's tissue, such as from the belly or back.

Mastectomy can have some side effects, including pain, edema, and reduced arm movement. Complications may potentially arise, such as infection, bleeding, and fluid accumulation. However, most women can recover successfully following the treatment and resume their normal activities with time and careful care.

Lymph Node Removal

Lymph node removal is a surgical technique that involves the removal of one or more lymph nodes from the body. This is often done as a part of the cancer treatment, especially if the malignancy has spread to the adjacent lymph nodes.

The lymph nodes are part of the body's immune system and help in battling infections and illnesses. They are little, bean-shaped structures that are present throughout the body, notably in the armpit, groin, neck, and chest.

During a lymph node removal surgery, the surgeon creates an incision in the skin and removes the afflicted lymph nodes. The number of lymph nodes removed will depend on the location and extent of the malignancy. In some circumstances, only one or a few lymph nodes may be removed, but in other cases, several lymph nodes may need to be removed. After the procedure, the excised lymph nodes are inspected under a microscope to detect if cancer cells are present.

Lymph node removal might cause some side effects, including discomfort, edema, and numbness in the affected area. It can also raise the risk of getting lymphedema, which is a disorder that causes swelling in the arm or leg owing to the accumulation of lymph fluid.

Breast cancer surgery is frequently conducted under general anesthesia, which means the patient will be sleeping during the process. The sort of surgery performed will depend on the size and location of the tumor, as well as the patient's personal preferences.

After breast cancer surgery, most patients will need to stay in the hospital for a short length of time to recover. Recovery time will vary based on the type of surgery performed, but most patients can return to their typical activities within a few weeks.

Breast cancer surgery may be followed by radiation therapy, chemotherapy, hormone therapy, targeted therapy, or a combination of these treatments. The particular treatment approach will rely on the individual patient's conditions

Radiation Therapy

Radiation therapy is a frequent treatment option for breast cancer that involves the use of high-energy radiation to eliminate cancer cells and decrease tumors. It is often used after surgery to remove malignant tissue to help lower the risk of cancer recurrence.

Radiation therapy works by destroying the DNA of cancer cells, which inhibits them from growing and dividing. It can be supplied externally using a machine called a linear accelerator, or internally through a radioactive source that is inserted inside the body near the malignant tissue.

External beam radiation therapy (EBRT) is the most prevalent type of radiation therapy used for breast cancer.

During EBRT, a machine delivers high-energy radiation to the breast from outside the body. Treatment is often provided daily for several weeks, with each session lasting only a few minutes.

Internal radiation therapy, also known as brachytherapy, involves the insertion of a radioactive source inside the breast near the malignant tissue. This type of radiation therapy is often utilized for tiny tumors and is provided over a shorter length of time than EBRT.

Radiation therapy can have some side effects, including exhaustion, skin irritation, and breast swelling. It can also increase the risk of acquiring other health concerns, including as heart disease and lung cancer, but these risks are normally minimal.

Chemotherapy

Chemotherapy is a treatment option for breast cancer that uses chemicals to kill cancer cells. Chemotherapy is primarily administered to individuals with invasive breast cancer, although it may also be used to treat some types of non-invasive breast cancer. Chemotherapy can be given before or after surgery, or in certain circumstances, it may be the primary treatment if surgery is not a possibility. Chemotherapy medications are normally given intravenously, however some can be taken orally. The medications circulate through the circulation and target cancer cells throughout the body. Chemotherapy may produce adverse effects, including hair loss, nausea, vomiting, exhaustion, and increased risk of infection. However, these adverse effects can often be treated with medicine and other supporting measures.

Hormone Treatment

Hormone therapy is a treatment option for breast cancer that is used to prevent the effects of hormones, such as estrogen and progesterone, on breast cancer cells. Hormone therapy is often used to treat hormone receptor-positive breast cancer, which indicates that the cancer cells contain receptors for estrogen and/or progesterone on their surface.

There are various different forms of hormone treatment medications, including selective estrogen receptor modulators (SERMs), aromatase inhibitors, and estrogen receptor downregulators (ERDs). SERMs, such as tamoxifen, act by inhibiting the effects of estrogen on breast cancer cells. Aromatase inhibitors, such as anastrozole and letrozole, act by preventing the production of estrogen in the body. ERDs, such as fulvestrant, act by inhibiting the estrogen receptor and causing it to break down.

Hormone therapy may be given before or after surgery, and it may also be used in combination with other treatments, such as chemotherapy or radiation therapy. The length of treatment will depend on the stage and kind of breast cancer, as well as the patient's overall condition.

Hormone therapy may cause adverse effects, including hot flashes, vaginal dryness, mood changes, and increased risk of blood clots. However, these adverse effects can often be treated with medicine and other supporting measures.

Targeted Therapy

Targeted therapy is a type of treatment for breast cancer that targets specific proteins or genes that are important in the growth and spread of cancer cells. Targeted therapy medications are meant to specifically target cancer cells and spare healthy cells, which can lower the risk of side effects compared to chemotherapy.

There are various distinct types of targeted therapy medications used to treat breast cancer, including:

- HER2-targeted therapy

HER2 is a protein that is overexpressed in some kinds of breast cancer. HER2-targeted treatment medicines, such as trastuzumab and pertuzumab, act by inhibiting the HER2 protein and decreasing the growth and spread of cancer cells.

- CDK4/6 inhibitors

CDK4/6 inhibitors, such as palbociclib, ribociclib, and abemaciclib, function by suppressing the activity of two proteins, CDK4 and CDK6, which are implicated in the growth and division of cancer cells. CDK4/6 inhibitors are used for the treatment of hormone receptor-positive, HER2-negative breast cancer.

- PARP inhibitors

PARP inhibitors, such as olaparib and talazoparib, function by limiting the action of an enzyme called PARP, which is involved in repairing damaged DNA. PARP inhibitors are used to treat breast cancer with BRCA mutations, which are genetic mutations that raise the risk of breast cancer.

Targeted therapy may be given alone or in combination with other treatments, such as chemotherapy or hormone therapy. The length of treatment will depend on the stage and kind of breast cancer, as well as the patient's overall condition.

Targeted therapy may induce side effects, including nausea, exhaustion, and increased risk of infection. However, these adverse effects can often be treated with medicine and other supporting measures.

Immunotherapy

Immunotherapy is a sort of cancer treatment that helps the body's immune system combat cancer cells. It works by either boosting the immune system to target cancer cells or by inhibiting the signals that cancer cells use to elude the immune system.

While immunotherapy has been beneficial in treating other types of cancer, it has not yet been widely used for breast cancer. However, there are current clinical trials evaluating the use of immunotherapy for breast cancer, notably for triple-negative breast cancer (TNBC), which is a subtype of breast cancer that is more difficult to treat.

One option being researched is the use of immune checkpoint inhibitors, which are medications that disrupt the signals that cancer cells use to elude the immune system. These medications have been beneficial in treating other forms of cancer, such as melanoma and lung cancer, and have showed promise in early clinical trials for TNBC.

Another option being researched is the use of CAR-T cell therapy, which is a sort of immunotherapy that involves extracting immune cells from a patient's blood, altering them in a laboratory to single out cancer cells, and then implanting them back into the patient's body. This technique has shown potential in early clinical studies for TNBC.

Chapter Five

COPING WITH BREAST CANCER

MANAGING SYMPTOMS

Talk To Your Doctor

- Prepare questions. Before you talk to your doctor about your breast cancer, it's vital to be prepared with certain questions. It can be beneficial to jot down these questions so that you don't forget them throughout the chat.

- Make sure to chat about your treatment options. Ask your doctor what your treatment options are and how they will effect your life. Make sure to discuss both the prospective benefits and side effects of each treatment, so you can make an informed decision.

- Talk about your feelings. It's vital to be open and honest with your doctor about how you are feeling and ask for help if needed. Your doctor can offer you with tools and ideas to help you manage with the changes that come with cancer treatment.

- Follow up. Make sure to follow up with your doctor after your conversation. If you still have questions, make sure to bring them up and ask it. Additionally, it can be good to take notes on the information provided, so you can refer to it later.

Take Care Of Yourself

Taking care of yourself might be just as vital as any other element of coping with breast cancer. There are a few easy things you can do to take care of yourself.

- Set aside time for yourself. This might be as simple as taking some time each day to do something that offers you joy — a few minutes of journaling, reading, or meditating. Making sure you maintain a healthy balance between rest and activity will assist too.
- Eat nutritious, balanced meals. Make sure you obtain enough of fresh fruits and vegetables, lean proteins, complex carbohydrates, and healthy fats. Eating nutrient-dense foods can assist to ease fatigue, enhance your energy, and improve your overall wellbeing.
- Stay active. Regular mild movement or exercise can help increase your mood, reduce some of the physical consequences of cancer and treatments, and can help keep your mind bright.

Manage Stress

Managing stress is a key aspect in managing with breast cancer. Common stresses connected with a breast cancer diagnosis can include fear of cancer recurrence, financial obligations, and emotional discomfort. As such, it is crucial to pursue appropriate ways of controlling stress in order to cope with the problems connected with breast cancer.

Here are a few ideas on how to manage stress with a breast cancer diagnosis:

- Take Time for Yourself: Take vacations from cancer-related activities, such as doctor visits and care treatments, and clear your schedule so that you can focus on things that offer you joy and happiness. Get a massage, read a book, or spend time doing the activities and hobbies that make you feel calm.
- Seek Support: Connect with family, friends, and other people who have been impacted by cancer in order to obtain support and to share experiences. Talking to those who may relate can help alleviate emotions of isolation, dread, and worry.
- Exercise: Exercise not only can assist reduce stress, but can also lessen physical symptoms and exhaustion. Start slow and progressively increase intensity as your body allows.

- Meditate: Practice meditation, mindfulness, and deep breathing to relax and to reduce stress.

By reducing stress, you can enhance your quality of life with a breast cancer diagnosis and find strength and comfort during this tough time.

Address Pains and Other Physical Symptoms

Pain management is a crucial aspect of coping with a diagnosis of breast cancer. Pain can be induced by several events, including surgery, radiation therapy and systemic chemotherapy. While various pain medications are available to assist manage pain, there are other lifestyle adjustments that can help decrease pain and other physical symptoms of breast cancer.

- Exercise: Exercise can help alleviate discomfort, strengthen the muscles around a tumor site, improve posture, and build up stamina. Incorporate hobbies like walking, swimming, yoga, or Tai Chi into your regular regimen.
- Get Enough Rest: Adequate rest is vital to help your body repair and cope with the physical effects of cancer therapy. Make sure

you get enough sleep, especially if you're getting chemotherapy.

- Stress Relief: Stress can increase back pain, headaches, exhaustion and other physical symptoms related with breast cancer. Relaxation techniques such as meditation, progressive relaxation, or self-hypnosis can assist relieve stress.

- Maintain a Healthy Diet: Consuming nourishing meals will aid in the fight against weariness and make it simpler to deal with the negative effects of cancer therapies.

- Speak To Someone: Discussing your physical and emotional needs with a friend, family member, or healthcare provider can frequently assist lessen the burden of cancer. If you feel the need to talk to someone, think about attending a support group for those who have breast cancer or seeking out a therapist.

Look Into Complementary Therapies

Many patients are now turning to alternative medicine to enhance or even replace conventional treatments for breast cancer, even though conventional therapies like surgery, chemotherapy, and radiation remain the main recommendations. Herbal treatments, acupuncture, meditation, and yoga are examples of alternative medicine that may provide useful extra tools for managing breast cancer and its symptoms.

To maintain and boost natural immunity, lower the toxic burden of radiation or chemotherapy, and treat common side effects including nausea, lack of appetite, anxiety, or depression, herbal treatments are employed.

Additionally, acupuncture can help to improve comfort, balance hormones, lower pain, and lessen anxiety and sadness.

Meditation, yoga, and tai chi are examples of mind-body exercises that can aid with stress management, mood enhancement, and relaxation. Additionally, they can boost energy and lessen fatigue, which will help with treatment-related lethargy. These techniques are proven to enhance the general quality of life and can help lower the likelihood of relapse following treatment.

To complement or replace a traditional treatment strategy, it may be beneficial to investigate the potential benefits of alternative medicine for breast cancer and accompanying symptoms. To ensure the safe and efficient use of alternative treatments, proper consultation and coordination with practitioners of both conventional and alternative medicine are essential.

Control Depression and Anxiety

- Educate Yourself: Learn all you can about depression and anxiety. You will be better able to control these illnesses the more you comprehend them. Spend some time reading, talking to an expert, or conducting online research.
- Track Symptoms: Record your symptoms of anxiety and depression. Make notes about your emotions, sleeping patterns, anxiety levels, and other pertinent details. By doing this, you may evaluate your development and choose the most effective symptom management techniques.

- Identify Triggers: It's critical to understand what makes you anxious or depressed. Understanding what causes depressive or panicky symptoms might help you better control your emotions.
- Practice relaxation: Discover relaxation methods that are effective for you and use

them frequently. You can manage stress and anxiety by practicing yoga, deep breathing, and mindfulness.

- Seek Professional treatment: If your emotions start to interfere with your daily tasks or become too overpowering, get professional treatment. You can develop a tailored strategy for controlling your anxiety and depression with the assistance of a therapist or psychiatrist.

- Seek Support: Make connections with those who have gone through similar experiences. A breast cancer support group or forum can offer priceless knowledge and solace. Although talking about your feelings isn't always easy, knowing you're not alone can be quite beneficial.

Establishing a Support System

While coping with one of life's greatest struggles, finding a breast cancer support network can be a terrific way to find solace, understanding, and knowledge. Patients, survivors, and carers have access to a variety of options, including support groups, internet chat rooms, and other organizations that specialize in offering assistance.

Speaking with a doctor or other medical expert is the first step in locating a breast cancer support group. They might have knowledge of neighborhood services, including support groups and planned activities. Additionally, friends and family can be a great resource for learning about support systems.

Finding breast cancer support groups is quite easy because of the Internet. Numerous national organizations offer online discussion boards, chat rooms, and directories of regional resources. These websites help learn about available treatments and research.

Events and support groups for those impacted by breast cancer are frequently listed in local newspapers, community bulletin boards, hospitals, and libraries. Meetings of support groups can be a terrific place to meet others who have similar experiences. A secure environment to ask concerns, give and receive emotional support, and build enduring relationships with other survivors can all be found in support groups.

Finally, it's critical to realize that support is accessible on a variety of levels. Those dealing with a breast cancer diagnosis can find support by talking to friends and family, attending a support group, getting one-on-one counseling, and using online resources.

Keeping Well-Being

Keeping healthy can play a significant role in coping with a breast cancer diagnosis. You may have greater control over your diagnosis and lessen the negative effects it has on your body and quality of life by taking care of your physical and emotional health.

Here are some pointers to help you stay healthy as you deal with breast cancer:

- Remain engaged.

One of the most crucial things to do to deal with cancer is to continue to be active. Cancer patients have a special chance to control their physical and mental health by engaging in physical activity. Exercise is a fantastic method to improve quality of life, manage stress and exhaustion, and reduce worry.

Cancer survivors are advised by the American Cancer Society to divide their exercises into two distinct components: aerobic (or aerobic-like) activity and resistance/strength training. Exercises like jogging and walking are aerobic activities that help burn calories and improve cardiovascular health. Exercises that involve resistance, such as weight-bearing exercises, elastic band exercises, or modest weights, can help maintain bone and muscular strength while reducing bone loss brought on by cancer therapies.

In addition to promoting physical health, research has shown that physical activity can help safeguard mental health. Exercise can assist enhance sleep and reduce stress and anxiety. It can create a sense of accomplishment to help people feel better about themselves.

If dealing with cancer, talk to your doctor before commencing any physical activity program. The doctor can provide recommendations on what type and level of activity is safe for you. Remember to start slow, and then gradually work up to 30 or more minutes of physical activity a day. It's crucial to be active, and it opens the chance of a more full remission.

Stay Connected

- Connect with other survivors: Being among individuals who can relate to your story can be immensely healing. Connecting with a support group can offer you a secure area to ask about concerns and discuss subjects that can be sensitive for you.

- Connect with friends and family: Lean on your support network, whether it be family or friends to help you through the trip. Your loved ones can do anything from lending a shoulder to cry on to practical aid like bringing groceries or transportation.
- Connect with professionals: Building a good relationship with your healthcare staff can help reduce any fears about breast cancer. They understand the process and can help you with solutions and guidance tailored to your needs.

- Connect with nature: Taking the time to walk outside and admire the environment can be wonderful for your emotional well-being. Take a peaceful walk, or try mind-body practices like yoga and meditation to help connect with your physical and spiritual self.
- Connect with yourself: Most importantly, give yourself time and permission to check in with your feelings. Take a few moments to

focus on your ideas, feelings, and of course, be kind to yourself.

Maintain A Healthy Diet

Eating a balanced diet is an important aspect of managing cancer. A good diet can help you stay energized and maintain a healthy weight, strengthen your immunity, and help you manage symptoms of cancer and treatment side effects.

- Eat a Variety of Foods: Including fruits, vegetables, whole grains, lean protein sources, low-fat dairy, and healthy fats in your diet. Fruits and vegetables are especially beneficial because of their antioxidant content. Eating a variety of foods gives all of the vital vitamins, minerals, and other nutrients your body needs to keep healthy and powerful.

- Avoid or Limit Processed Foods: Processed foods generally contain saturated fats, added sugar, and sodium, which can be unhealthy. Try to avoid or minimize processed foods such as chips and candy.

- Making Healthy Beverage Choices: Limit sugary drinks and drink lots of water. On occasion, herbal teas, green tea, and other low-sugar beverages can be consumed.

- Moderation: Eating smaller meals more frequently throughout the day will keep your blood sugar constant and help your body metabolize food effectively.
- Pay Attention to Nutrients: Eating foods that are abundant in nutrients like vitamins, minerals, and antioxidants will improve your immune system and help your body fight and prevent cancer. Some instances include:
- Leafy greens like spinach and kale, Vegetables like broccoli and carrots.

By following the above methods, you may ensure that you are maintaining a nutritious diet to cope with cancer. Be sure to see a doctor or you will get the essential nutrients your body needs to fight cancer and stay healthy.

Get Adequate Sleep.

Getting enough sleep when you're living with breast cancer is vital for preserving your emotional and physical health. Good sleep helps you manage stress, enhance your immune system, and improve your general well-being.

Start by ensuring that your sleeping environment is comfortable and conducive to receiving quality sleep. Make sure that your bedroom is dark, quiet, and free from distractions. Make sure that your bedding is comfortable and keep a cool room temperature. If you're disturbed by outside noise or light, attempt to use earplugs or an eye mask.

Also, develop a regular sleeping routine and create healthy sleeping habits. Always try to go to bed and wake up at the same time each day. Avoid drinking caffeine or eating a substantial meal too late at night. Also, avoid using your phone, computer, or other technology in bed. You can also try to relax before bed with deep breathing, meditation, or yoga.

Finally, make sure to talk to your doctor if you are having chronic difficulties sleeping. They may be able to recommend therapies such as cognitive-behavioral therapy or sleep medicines if necessary.

Chapter Six

PREVENTION OF CANCER

Maintain a Healthy Weight

- Eat a balanced diet with plenty of fruits, vegetables, lean proteins, and whole grains.
- Reduce foods and drinks that are heavy in sugar, salt, and harmful fats.
- Exercise regularly to help preserve a healthy weight.
- If you are pre-menopausal, consider taking steps to decrease your exposure to estrogen-like substances (xenoestrogens) in the environment.
- Reduce stress levels with relaxation techniques and awareness.

Avoid Alcohol

Drinking of alcohol has been related to an increased risk of breast cancer. Even moderate levels of drinking, such as two alcoholic beverages per day, have been connected with an elevated risk. Therefore, to lower the risk of breast cancer, it is recommended to limit or prevent alcohol use.

There are numerous measures that can be taken to avoid alcohol and minimize the risk of breast cancer. First, individuals should be conscious of their drinking patterns and take action to limit intake. This can include tracking one's intake, preparing ahead to not have access to alcohol, or avoiding social gatherings where drinking may occur. Additionally, drinking patterns can be modified by substituting non-alcoholic drinks, such as juice or soda, for alcoholic beverages. Finally, individuals should be aware of the health dangers involved with drinking and take the time to educate themselves on the ramifications of alcohol usage.

Limit Hormone Replacement Therapy

Hormone replacement therapy (HRT) is a method of treatment that replaces hormones that are lost during menopause. It has also been used to treat a variety of other ailments, including hot flashes, vaginal dryness, and night sweats. While HRT can help with many of these symptoms, it may also increase the chance of certain types of cancer, including breast cancer.

For this reason, many healthcare experts advocate restricting hormone replacement medication to prevent breast cancer. The choice to use HRT should only be made after a careful examination of the potential dangers and benefits. Women who are at a higher risk for developing breast cancer due to their age, family history, or other factors should be extremely cautious while using HRT.

Get Screened

Getting checked periodically for breast cancer is one of the most critical things a woman can do to preserve her long-term health. Regular screenings can help discover any risk factors for breast cancer early on, so it's crucial to make sure that you and your healthcare provider create a strategy to monitor your breast health.

Screenings include mammograms (x-rays of the breast tissue that can detect any irregularities in the size and shape of the breast tissue), ultrasounds (high-frequency sound waves used to check for solid masses), and clinical breast exams (where your doctor physically checks your breast tissue for any abnormalities).

These tests can help detect small changes in breast tissue before they are evident to the naked eye. If something is identified, further testing like biopsies may be arranged to evaluate if the regions are malignant. Detectinng breast cancer early is very crucial because it aids to successfully treat the cancer.

Breastfeed

Breastfeeding can be an effective approach to minimize your chance of developing breast cancer later in life. Breastfeeding releases hormones and other chemicals that can help to protect the breasts from damage that could lead to cancer. This protective effect is the strongest when women breastfeed for at least six months and typically up to two years. Studies have revealed that women who breastfeed had up to a 25% decreased chance of having breast cancer compared with women who didn't breastfeed. This finding is especially true for mothers who breastfeed longer than six months.

Avoid Unnecessary Radiation Exposure

Radiation exposure is an established risk factor for cancer. While some radiation exposure is unavoidable in our daily lives, there are steps you may do to lower your chance of acquiring cancer from radiation exposure.

- Limit unnecessary medical imaging: Medical imaging examinations such as X-rays, CT scans, and PET scans involve ionizing radiation, which might increase your risk of cancer over time. While these tests can be essential for identifying and treating medical disorders, it is vital to limit unneeded imaging tests and to only have them when indicated by your healthcare professional.

- Protect yourself from the sun: Ultraviolet (UV) radiation from the sun can cause skin cancer. To protect yourself, wear protective gear, use sunscreen with an SPF of at least 30, and avoid outside activities during high solar hours.

- Avoid radon exposure: Radon is a naturally occurring gas that can infiltrate homes and buildings and raise the risk of lung cancer. To decrease your radon exposure, have your house tested for radon and take steps to mitigate radon levels if necessary.

- Be mindful of occupational radiation exposure: Certain occupations, such as healthcare professionals and nuclear power plant workers, may be at elevated risk of radiation exposure. If you work in an occupation that includes radiation exposure, be sure to follow safety requirements and wear protective equipment when necessary.

- Choose non-ionizing radiation alternatives: Non-ionizing radiation, such as radio waves and microwaves, is generally regarded as safe. When possible, seek non-ionizing radiation alternatives, such as utilizing a landline phone instead of a cell phone or using an ultrasound instead of an X-ray.

Eat a Balanced Diet

A balanced diet is vital for overall health, and new research has revealed that it may be especially useful for preventing breast cancer. Eating a balanced diet, made of a range of foods from different food categories, can assist to ensure that the body receives all the required vitamins, minerals, and other nutrients it needs to keep it healthy.

Fruits and vegetables are especially significant for their cancer-fighting antioxidant and anti-inflammatory capabilities. Dark leafy greens, especially cruciferous vegetables like broccoli, Brussels sprouts, and cauliflower, are high in potent antioxidants and phytochemicals that can aid to reduce inflammation in the body, activating or increasing the body's natural defense mechanism.

Whole grains in the diet are also advantageous as they include lignans, substances with antioxidant and anti-inflammatory effects that may reduce the incidence of breast cancer. Legumes are also a good source of fiber, protein, and other key nutrients that support general health and protect against breast cancer.

A diet should also contain quality sources of protein such as fish, beans, almonds, and eggs. These meals have cholesterol-lowering effects and also provide the body with vital omega-3 fatty acids, which possess anti-inflammatory characteristics that can help reduce the

Be Physically Active

Physical activity helps decrease cholesterol and insulin levels. It can also help you maintain a healthy weight, which can lessen your risk of certain types of cancer. Aim for at least 30 minutes of moderate to strenuous activity every day.

MEDICATIONS FOR CANCER PREVENTION

Numerous drugs may be used to help prevent breast cancer in certain women who are at high risk of developing the disease. These drugs operate by limiting the effects of estrogen, a hormone that can accelerate the growth of some breast tumors.

Here are some drugs used for avoiding breast cancer:

- Tamoxifen

Tamoxifen is a medicine that is often used to treat breast cancer, but it can also be used to prevent breast cancer in women who are at high risk of developing the disease. Tamoxifen is a selective estrogen receptor modulator (SERM) that suppresses the effects of estrogen in breast tissue.

- Raloxifen

Raloxifene is another SERM that is used to prevent breast cancer in postmenopausal women who are at high risk of getting the disease. Like tamoxifen, raloxifene prevents the actions of estrogen in breast tissue.

- Aromatase inhibitors

Aromatase inhibitors are a class of drugs that suppress the production of estrogen in postmenopausal women. These drugs may be used to prevent breast cancer in women who are at high risk of developing the illness.

  - Exemestane: Exemestane is an aromatase inhibitor that is used to prevent breast cancer in postmenopausal women who are at high risk of getting the disease.

- Calcium and vitamin D supplements can help reduce the incidence of breast cancer in pre- and postmenopausal women.

It is crucial to note that some medications can have adverse effects and are not fit for everyone. Your healthcare practitioner can assist assess if these medications are appropriate for you based on your unique risk factors and medical history. Additionally, it is vital to continue to follow established screening guidelines for breast cancer detection, even if you are taking drugs to prevent the disease.

Chapter Seven

RESOURCES FOR BREAST CANCER

Organizations and Groups

There are several organizations and organizations committed to breast cancer research, education, and support. Here are some of the key organizations and groups for breast cancer:

- Susan G. Komen:

Susan G. Komen is one of the largest breast cancer organizations in the world, dedicated to supporting research, offering information and support, and campaigning for breast cancer patients and survivors.

- National Breast Cancer Foundation

The National Breast Cancer Foundation is a nonprofit organization that provides education and support for breast cancer patients and their families, as well as funding for breast cancer research.

- Breast Cancer Research Foundation

The Breast Cancer Research Foundation is a nonprofit organization that funds breast cancer research around the world, with an emphasis on finding a cure for the disease.

- Young Survival Coalition

The Young Survival Coalition is a nonprofit organization dedicated to providing support and services for young women with breast cancer, as well as campaigning for their special needs.

- Living Beyond Breast Cancer

Living Beyond Breast Cancer is a nonprofit organization that provides education and support for breast cancer patients and survivors, as well as their families and healthcare providers.

- American Cancer Society

The American Cancer Society is a nonprofit organization that provides education, support, and resources for all types of cancer, including breast cancer.

These foundations and organizations can provide useful resources, support, and information for breast cancer patients and their families.

Breast Cancer Research

Breast cancer research is an ongoing field of study that strives to better understand the causes of breast cancer, find novel treatments, and enhance the lives of those impacted by the disease. Breast cancer is the most frequent cancer among women globally, and scientific efforts have led to substantial advances in the diagnosis and treatment of the illness.

One field of breast cancer research involves researching the genetic abnormalities that can increase a person's chance of developing the disease. Researchers have found many genes, such as BRCA1 and BRCA2, that are connected with an elevated risk of developing breast cancer. Understanding these genetic variants can assist identify individuals who may be at higher risk of getting breast cancer and enable clinicians to deliver more targeted screening and preventative efforts.

Another area of study involves developing novel and improved treatments for breast cancer. Chemotherapy, radiation therapy, and surgery are now the primary treatments for breast cancer, but researchers are studying new approaches, such as targeted therapy and immunotherapy, that can more effectively target cancer cells while minimizing adverse effects.

In addition to discovering novel medicines, researchers are also aiming to improve the quality of life for breast cancer survivors. This includes establishing techniques to handle the physical and mental adverse effects of treatment, such as exhaustion, discomfort, and anxiety.

Breast cancer research is a collaborative effort including scientists, doctors, patients, and advocacy. Funding for breast cancer research comes from a range of sources, including government grants, private organizations, and donations from individuals and corporations.

Overall, breast cancer research is an important field of study that has led to substantial breakthroughs in the prevention, detection, and treatment of breast cancer. Ongoing research efforts show promise for further improving outcomes for persons affected by this disease.

CONCLUSION

Breast cancer is a complex disease that can impact anyone, regardless of age, gender, or race. It is the most frequent cancer among women globally and is caused by a mix of genetic, environmental, and lifestyle factors.

However, there is hope for people impacted by breast cancer. Advances in screening, diagnosis, and therapy have considerably improved outcomes for patients, and ongoing research initiatives offer promise for further enhancing these results.

Prevention is equally crucial in the fight against breast cancer. Maintaining a healthy lifestyle, such as eating a balanced diet and exercising regularly, can help minimize the risk of developing breast cancer. Regular tests, such as mammograms, can also help discover breast cancer early when it is most curable.

For those impacted by breast cancer, there is a range of resources available for support and care. assistance groups, counseling, and other services can give emotional and practical assistance to patients and their families.

There are numerous steps that can be performed to promote change in the fight against breast cancer:

- Improve awareness: One of the most critical stages in the fight against breast cancer is to improve awareness about the disease. This can be done through public education campaigns, social media outreach, and community activities.
- Advocate for research funding: Research is vital to identifying new treatments and improving outcomes for those afflicted by breast cancer. Advocating for additional research funding can assist speed advances in the fight against the disease.
- Support patients and survivors: Breast cancer can have a tremendous impact on patients and their families. Supporting persons affected by breast cancer through advocacy, counseling, and other services can help improve their quality of life.

- Promote healthy lifestyles: Maintaining a healthy lifestyle, such as eating a balanced diet and exercising regularly, can help minimize the risk of developing breast cancer. Promoting healthy behaviors in communities can help prevent the disease.
- Remove barriers to care: Access to quality care is crucial for breast cancer patients. Removing barriers to care, such as financial or geographic constraints, can assist guarantee that patients receive the care they need.
- Foster collaboration: The fight against breast cancer requires collaboration among researchers, healthcare providers, patients, and advocates. Fostering collaboration can assist accelerate progress and guarantee that all stakeholders are working together towards a single goal.

By implementing these actions, we can drive change in the battle against breast cancer and improve outcomes for people afflicted by the disease.

In conclusion, breast cancer is a serious disease that demands constant care and study. However, with the correct resources and support, it is feasible to lessen

the effect of breast cancer and improve outcomes for
those impacted by this disease.